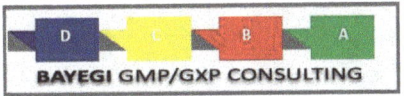

www. Bayegi.com

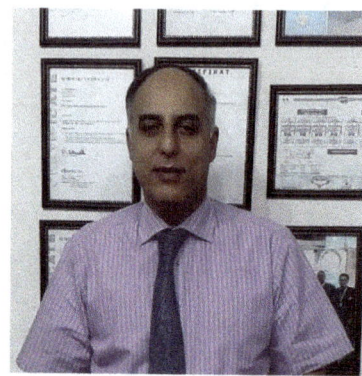

With over 15 years of experience in the pharmaceutical industry and successful implementation of numerous GMP projects, the author brings extensive knowledge and experience to this book.

E-Mail: contact@bayegi.com

www.bayegi.com

Parviz Bayegi

FMEA fast & professional for GMP projects

Step-by-step learning with colored content, templates and case studies

Pharmacy/Biotech/ATMP/Medical-Device/QM (Quality Management)

Foreword

Failure Mode and Effects Analysis (FMEA) is a structured process for identifying potential risks and defects of a product or process. This can be used during the development phase, but also during any update or evaluation.

In the quality assurance of sterile production in the pharmaceutical industry, one is forced to analyze every risk area/process. Precisely because of the new EU-GMP Annex 1 of 2022, QA specialists are forced to evaluate more processes according to contamination risk. Through the FMEA, the risks can be defined very quickly and a measure can be determined as required.

In order to be able to convey FMEA quickly and professionally, the skin characteristics in this book have been placed on practical topics and examples.

The book is excellently suited for all those who want to carry out an FMEA quickly and professionally without much prior knowledge.

Have fun and congratulations for your project

Your Parviz Bayegi

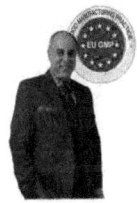

Table of contents

What is FMEA?

Failure Mode and Impact Analysis (FMEA) is a method that allows companies to anticipate failures in the design phase by identifying all possible defects in a design or manufacturing process. FMEA is a risk analysis method developed by NASA during the Apollo program. In various phases of further development, FMEA has undergone significant improvements through application in the automotive and mechanical engineering industries, as well as in the semiconductor and microelectronics industries. These applications demonstrate the versatility of the method. The FMEA is considered the most frequently practiced form of risk analysis and an important document for the preparation of qualification measures such as SAT/FAT, IQ, OQ, PQ.

FMEA is a preventive method that enables a quantitative assessment of errors and their possible causes in terms of probability of occurrence, severity of the error and probability of detection.

Illustration 1: the three criteria for assessing possible risks

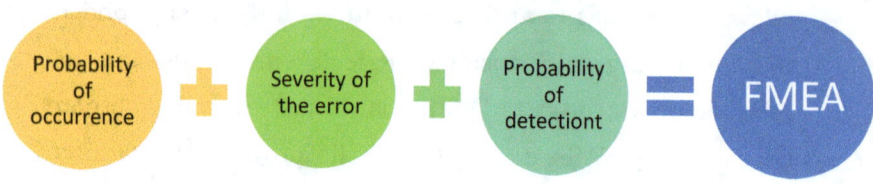

The essence is that the execution of the FMEA is based on the understanding of the product and the process. This means that FMEA cannot be carried out without appropriate preparation (e.g. process descriptions).

In the ICH Q9 guideline (Quality risk management), the FMEA is described as follows:

"FMEA (see IEC 60812) provides an assessment of potential failure modes for processes and their likely impact on results and/or product performance. Once failure modes are established, risk mitigation can be used to eliminate, contain, reduce, or control the potential for failure. FMEA is based on product and process understanding. The FMEA methodically divides the analysis of complex processes into manageable steps. It is a powerful tool for summarizing the important failure modes, failure causes, probabilities, and error impacts."

1. Objectives and areas of application

From the objectives mentioned below, we can conclude that FMEA is generally not created as a one-time procedure during the implementation of processes and/or facilities, but that FMEA needs to be constantly adapted in case changes are made to processes/facilities. In the event of such changes, the FMEA can also serve as a basis for risk assessment.

The objectives of an FMEA are as follows:

- The preventive identification and evaluation of possible failures, their causes and consequences during the implementation phase of processes/facilities

- The preventive identification and evaluation of possible errors, their causes and consequences for possible changes to existing processes and/or facilities (ideally based on an existing FMEA from the implementation phase)

- Identification of measures to mitigate risk

- Avoidance or reduction of possible failures

- Increasing product quality

- Increased process stability

- Creation of a broad understanding of the process among employees

An FMEA can be applied or triggered in the following areas:

- New process

- Process changes

- New product

- Product changes

- New plant

- Changes to a facility

- Implementation of a new IT-system

- Changes to IT-systems

The creation of the FMEA should be carried out at the earliest possible stage, as an earlier implementation of the changes can still be quick and cost-effective.

2. FMEA Process Flow

FMEA will take place in a multi-stage process, with each stage being a prerequisite for the next.

Illustration No.2: FMEA Process flow

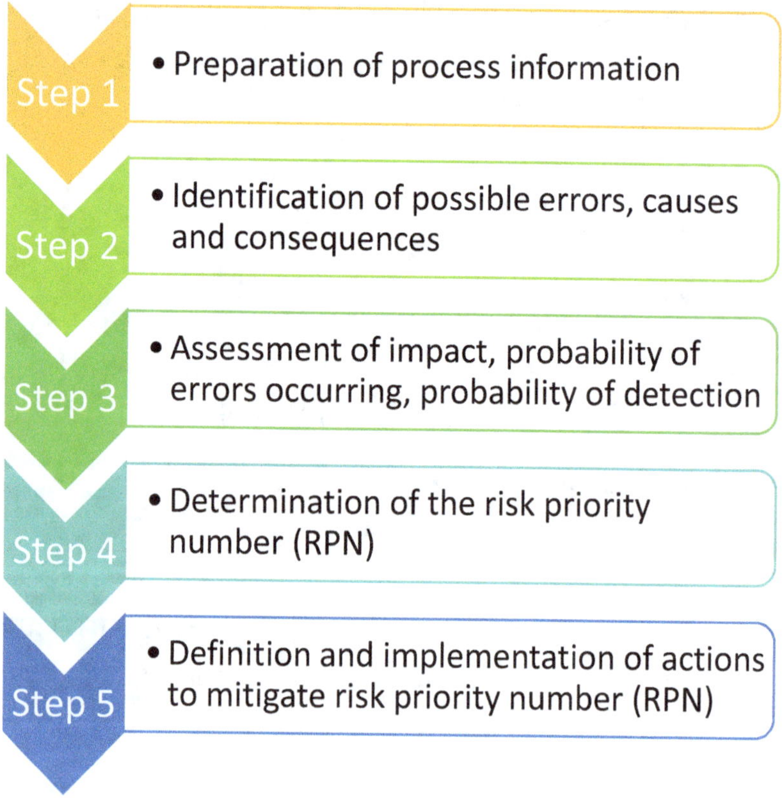

Step 1
- Preparation of process information

Step 2
- Identification of possible errors, causes and consequences

Step 3
- Assessment of impact, probability of errors occurring, probability of detection

Step 4
- Determination of the risk priority number (RPN)

Step 5
- Definition and implementation of actions to mitigate risk priority number (RPN)

3. Types of FMEA

There are also different FMEAs for different risk analyses. The structure and processes are the same for all FMEAs, only the source data is different. This source data can come from a project evaluation, process stage, or even a machine specification. In all FMEA types, the source data (requirements) are listed first. Then, these requirements are evaluated for possible/potential errors. In further steps, these errors are evaluated from the point of view of the impact of the errors, probability of the errors occurring, and detection of the errors. In the next step, measures are defined depending on the risk area. In the last step, the possible/potential errors are evaluated again after the measures have been carried out.

Illustration No.3: FMEA content

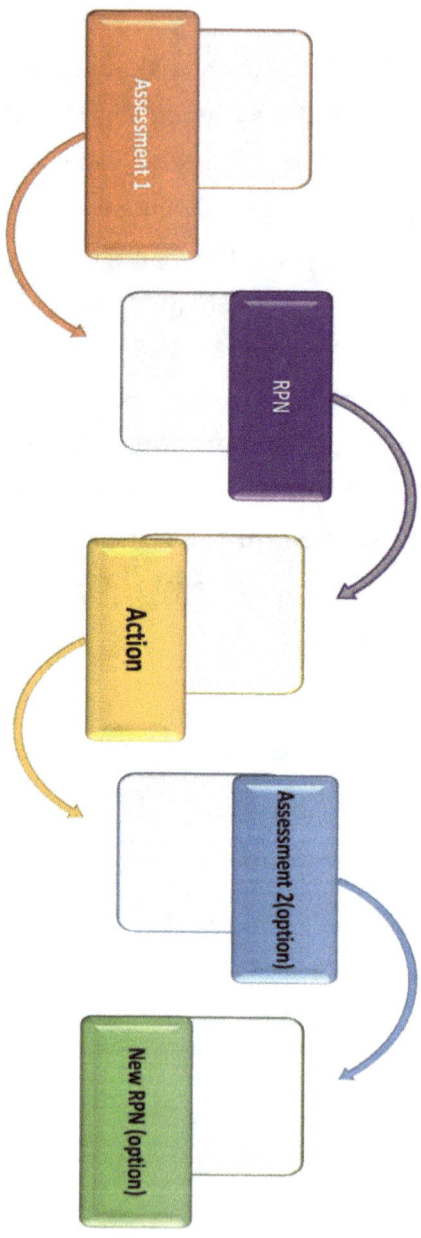

3.1 Project-FMEA

Before a project is carried out in the pharmaceutical industry, a project risk analysis should be prepared. This can be realized by means of a project FMEA. In a project FMEA, the project components (trades) are analysed and evaluated for risk.

Illustration No.4: Example of a Project-FMEA

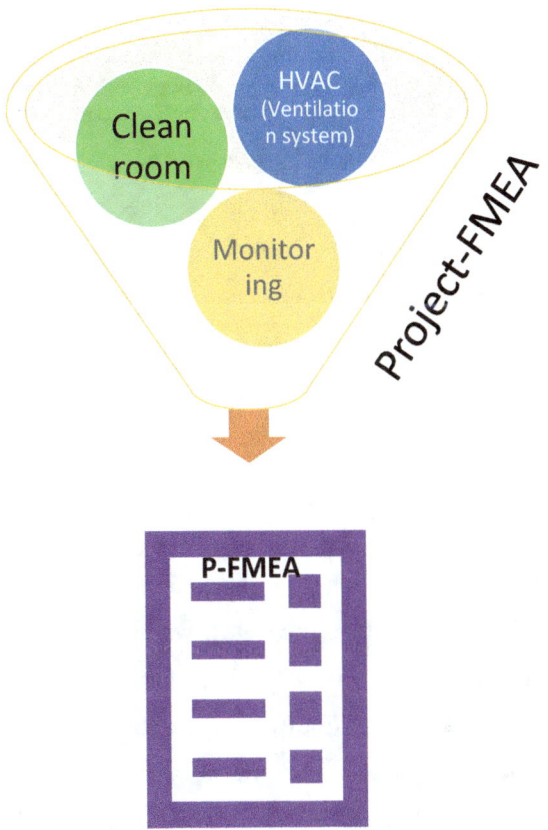

3.2 Design-FMEA

This FMEA is often prepared before the start of a project and before the strategies for validation are written. The design or construction FMEA is used in development and construction to assess the suitability of a product for production and assembly as early as possible and to prepare the project for the validation processes.

3.3 System-FMEA

In a System-FMEA, the focus is on the functions and relationships that are unique to the entire system (i.e., those that do not exist at lower levels). In addition to accounting for single-point failures (where a single component failure can lead to the complete failure of the entire system), System-FMEA includes failure modes associated with interfaces and interactions.

3.4 Hardware-/Equipment-FMEA

A Hardware-FMEA assesses the risks from the hardware and electronics sector. In a Hardware-FMEA, the focus is on analyzing hardware functions. In all pharmaceutical projects, a Hardware-/Equipment-FMEA is created, which is one of the most important components of the design qualifications (DQ). The points of user and technical requirements (URS/TRS) are components of the Hardware-/Equipment-FMEA. This means that each quality-relevant point from URS/TRS is analyzed and evaluated separately in the Hardware-/Equipment FMEA from the point of view of QMP/quality. Once possible errors have been identified, appropriate qualification measures such as FAT/SAT/IQ/OQ/PQ are entered for each point. This FMEA is the prerequisite for the subsequent qualification test. The Equipment-FMEA is not written until the respective URS/TRS are available.

Illustration No.5: Example of a Ventilation System (Equipment) FMEA

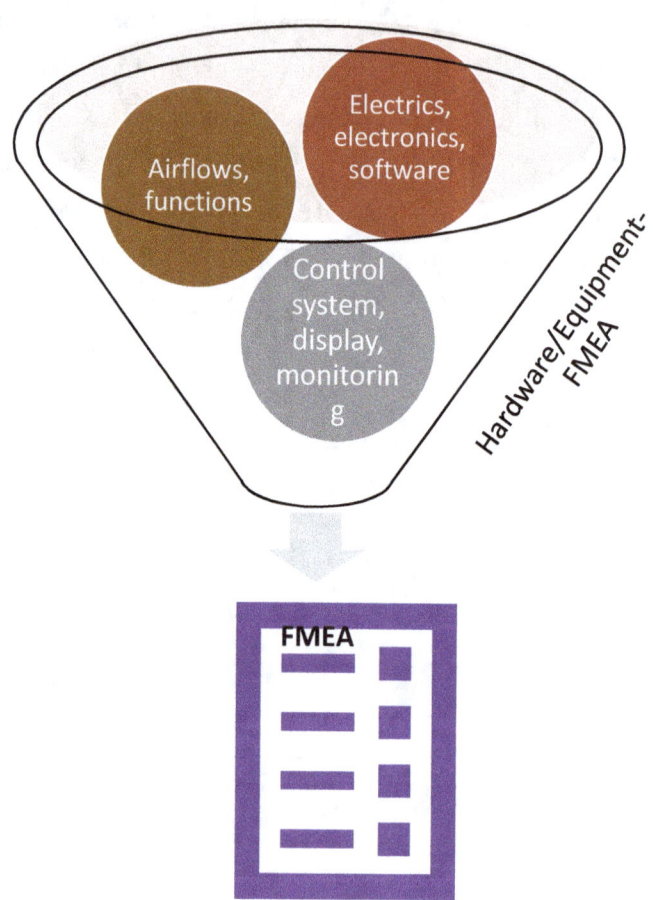

3.5 Software-FMEA

A Software-FMEA assesses the risks from the software sector and has the task of analysing and evaluating the generated program code. The small PC/display controllers for machines and systems are not evaluated by a software FMEA. Rather, it refers to the complete software system, for example an EWC system or a monitoring system for the monitoring of cleanrooms.

3.6 Process-FMEA

The main goal of a Process-FMEA is to identify the risk prior to manufacturing. Mitigating the identified risk prior to the approval process for the first item or product validates the expectation of superior process performance.

4. When should a FMEA be performed?

There are several reasons why it makes sense to perform a failure mode and impact analysis:

- When you're designing a new product, process or service

- If you plan to run an existing process in a different way

- If you have a quality improvement goal for a specific process

- When you need to understand and improve the flaws of a process

When identifying defects, it is important not to focus only on GMP-relevant errors. In practice, it has proven useful to include as many types of potential failures as possible (e.g. business risks, environmental risks, security risks, etc.).

Even though this means a greater amount of documentation at first (which is not essential for regulatory purposes), there are still many advantages. For example, the potential risks for business-critical processes should also be identified so that, if necessary, measures can also be defined to minimize non-GMP risks and thus make the processes more stable and reliable.

5. Preparation/Implementation of FMEA

To carry out a FMEA, all relevant process information must be available (project scope, user requirements/URS, requirement specifications, functional specifications, plans). First, the respective overall process structure should be displayed and then divided into further detailed subprocessing steps. The description is mainly used to map the process to be analyzed and its interfaces. In addition, the

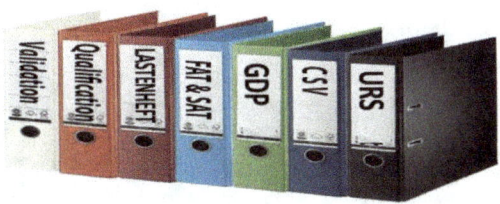

structuring of the processes at different levels allows classification according to the level of detail and possible influence.

Example: According to the user's requirements, the lines of sterilization units must be made of stainless steel. Now these points are included in the FMEA under:

10. ... Sterilization Unit/Tubes

10.1 ... Pilotages

10.1.1 ... Material made of stainless steel

Ideally, these descriptions should be in the form of process descriptions (e.g., flowcharts as shown in Illustration No., pp. 62,75). The individual process steps are assigned unique numbers to enable unambiguous referencing later.

5.1 Possible errors and consequences

Identifying possible errors, their consequences and causes of errors is the most time-consuming part of FMEA. Every single processing step is analyzed for possible errors at all levels. All kinds of

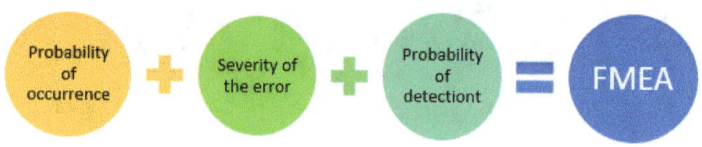

influencing factors such as machinery, labour, material, method and environment must be taken into account.

Errors that may seem hypothetical must also be considered, as the probability of occurrence is only taken into account at a later stage of the FMEA.

Especially in the initial phase of the execution of FMEAs, the identification of possible errors is very time-consuming. If several similar processes/facilities have already been analyzed, there may be similarities in the occurrence of errors and the effort required for this phase is reduced. However, this can be very time-consuming for a complex project. Therefore, in the case of a complex project, the FMEA is prepared by an expert with many years of experience.

After the FMEA draft has been prepared by experts, the FMEA draft is sent as a review to the interdisciplinary members from production, laboratory, quality assurance and engineering. This team evaluates the potential bugs and reports their suggestions as needed. Only after the FMEA has been identified and approved as a review by team members can a final FMEA be created.

Once all potential errors and consequences or causes of errors have been documented, they must be organized systematically. Many different causes of failure can often lead to the same error, while the same error can have different consequences. This is documented in a form to ensure traceability.

5.2 Risk assessment

The processes and the resulting possible errors are evaluated according to the following criteria:

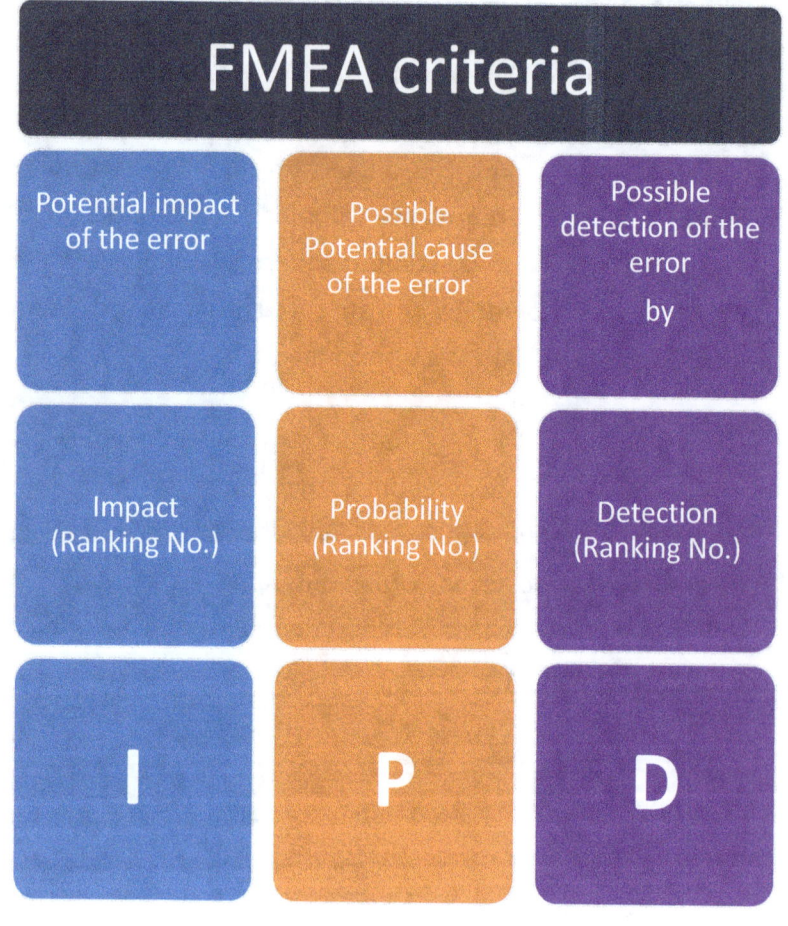

For each criterion (**I**, **P**, **D**), a table is created in which

- **Impact** Potential (Renking no.)

- **Probability** of error occurring (Renking no.)

- **Detection** of errors (Renking no.)

analysed and quantified.

Illustration No. 6: FMEA table for ranking **I**, **P**, **D**

Company Logo

Process FMEA case study

Lfd. Nr.	Function or malfunction requirement	Possible potential malfunction	Potential impact of the error	Impact (Ranking No.) **I**	Possible Potential cause of the error	Probability (Ranking No.) **P**	Possible detection of the error by	Detection (Ranking No.) **D**	RPN	Recommended action	Neu Auswirkung	Neu Wahrscheinlich-keit	Neu Erkennung	Neu RPN	Neue Risiko n identifiziert
1	Weighing process	E.g.: Quantities and weight deviations for raw materials	Formulation error, production stop	9	Scale not calibrated, error in weighing report,	5	By operators/Q C staff	7	315	Validated weighing process	9	3	1	27	Nicht nötig

28

5.3 Evaluation of errors/RPN

In the error evaluation phase, only one line in the FMEA form is usually evaluated at a time. For example, if there are multiple causes of errors listed in separate rows associated with an error, only those errors need to be considered individually. However, if the different causes of errors are combined in one row, the causes of errors are evaluated together.

The following aspects of errors are evaluated:

- Impact (Severity of Error Sequence) **(I)**

- Probability (Probability of Error) **(P)**

- Detection (Error Detection Probability) **(D)**

These three error characteristics are assigned numerical values (e.g. 1-10). The sum (number) of impact, probability, and detection results in the risk priority number (RPN).

Impact x **Probability** x **Detection** = **RPN**

It is important that these three assessments are conducted independently. For example, the assessment of the severity of an error must not include the likelihood of its occurrence or detection. The possible value ranges (scope of possible numerical values) of the individual error characteristics must be specifically defined by the company. Values from 1 to 10 can be allowed for each defect curve. When determining the possible ranges of values, it is always important to develop an FMEA valuation guideline before executing so that the significance of each numerical value is defined.

5.4 Impact of errors

The severity of an error is a key feature of this assessment. The severity of the error is generally determined by the consequences of the error. It should be clarified in advance whether the severity of the error only affects the "end user" (e.g. patients) or whether the severity of the error should be considered for the next "customer". The latter is usually the option, as it increases the stability of processes and minimizes the business risks that should be preferred (e.g. due to unusable products that need to be destroyed). The numerical value increases with increasing severity from 1-10 (see table below).

Table 1: Example of an Error Impact Assessment Guide

Impact of Error (I)		
Impact (examples)	**Classification**	**Ranking**
No adverse effects on product/process quality can be derived.	Insignificant	1
No adverse effects on product/process quality are expected.	Low	2
A usable product is to be expected. The master batch record is satisfied, although there are some variations in the process.	Low	3
A usable product is to be expected. The master batch record is satisfied, although there are significant variations in the	Low	4
The product is of limited use (specification is borderline), the process is stable.	Medium	5
The product can only be used to a limited extent (specification is borderline), there are slight deviations in the process.	Medium	6
The product can only be used to a limited extent (specification is borderline).	Medium	7
The product is unusable, damage to the health of patients must be eliminated.	High	8
The product is unusable, damage to the health of patients cannot be completely eliminated.	High	9
The product is unusable, harm to the patient's health is likely.	High	10

5.5 Probability of error

For a risk, it is of great importance to determine how often an error occurs or can occur. The more often an error occurs, the higher the risk. This means, for example, that W = 1 could stand for a rare occurrence and W = 10 for a very common occurrence. The probability of occurrence is usually determined by the cause of the error. For example, the probability of failure of sensors that are used on a daily basis.

Table 2: Example of an assessment guide for probability of error

Probability of error (P)		
Classification of probability	**Probable occurrence**	**Ranking**
Extremely likely	Very high	10
1 x per layer	Very high	9
1 x a day	High	8
1 x per week	High	7
1 x per month	Medium	6
1 x in 3 months	Medium	5
1 x in 6 months	Medium	4
1 x a year	Low	3
1 x in 3 years	Low	2
Very low	Low	1

5.6 Error detection

When determining risk, it is important to know whether a fault is detected by the factory employee, supplier, customer or consumer. The better the error can be detected, the lower the risk. Thus, the numerical value decreases from 10 to 1 the higher the probability of detection. This would mean that $E = 1$ is a value that can only be achieved, for example, if a fully automated 100% test is integrated into the process or production flow. Example: $E = 10$ means that no error is detected. This means that error detection is generally detected when the error has already been caused. In this case, there will be no surveillance.

Table 3: Example of an assessment guide for defect detection

Detection/Detection(D)		
Detection Type	**Discovery**	**Ranking**
The defect is detected in 100% of cases, e.g. by automatic measurements, strikingly likely	Very high	1
The error is detected in 100% of cases, e.g. by means of measurement protocols	High	2
The error is detected, e.g. due to error, the process is automatically stopped	High	3
The error is detected, e.g. by random check	High	4
The error is detected, e.g. by manual control	Medium	5
The fault is likely to be detected, e.g. by repair service	Medium	6
The fault can be detected, e.g. by manual control	Medium	7
The fault can be detected, e.g. by visual inspection	Low	8
The defect can be detected randomly, e.g. sporadic visual test	Low	9
The error can be detected visually by chance, strikingly unlikely	Very low	10

5.7 Rating RPN

Once the rankings for impact, probability and detection have been determined, the individual processes and functions are evaluated according to the specifications. I would like to explain this with an example: According to the specifications, a visual message (red light) should appear in the event of malfunctions from a filling machine that lead to a standstill. Now let's put this requirement in the FMEA table under the heading of the filling line. After that, we enter the possible malfunction in the table. For example, if there is a malfunction, no visual message is activated. From this malfunction, we create the possible ranking for impact, probability, and detection and enter the number into the table. The risk priority number RPN is calculated by multiplying the values A, W and E.

I x P x D = RPN

Using the valuation numbers described above, we get an RPN number = X. In addition to RPN, the company's own risk tolerance is also of great importance. At this level, the company sets the boundaries for defining actions.

The company needs to determine the RPN number, which is the critical level. The risk-mitigating measures are now being implemented. The risk-mitigating measures consist mostly of FAT/SAT protocols and IQ, OQ, PQ tests. If these measures are not sufficient, further risk-mitigating measures should be considered. These risk-mitigating measures are evaluated within the FMEA in two steps.

- Assessment prior to risk mitigation measures

- Assessment according to the risk mitigation measures (option)

The colors signal the conditions

Risk color		Ranking
conditions for	Risk Very Low	X
I, P, D	Risk Low	X
	Risk Medium	X
	Risk High	X
	Risk Very High	X

5.8 Rating RPN (first review)

If, in the first assessment (see p.61 template steps 1 to 11), the RPN number is higher than 130 or the impact ranking is higher than 7, measures must be taken to reduce the risk (see table below). These are the basic conditions for the initial assessment. You can set the numbers as you wish, depending on your imagination. For example, I use the number 130 as a limit. All RPNs above 130 are defined as a risk area and the risk must be mitigated by measures so that the RPN is set below 130 in the second assessment.

🔔 The number 130 is a fictitious number. The defined limit value is set by them. This can also be, for example, the RPN limit number 150. Accordingly, if RPN=150, the risk must be minimized by a measure.

A different structure/figures can be defined for each project/FMEA.

Please note that the calculation of the RPN Illustrations for the respective functions is only an assessment for the risk calculation and should only be carried out by GMP-technical specialists.

Table 4: Evaluation of RPN **before** the introduction of measures (e.g. IQ, OQ, PQ)

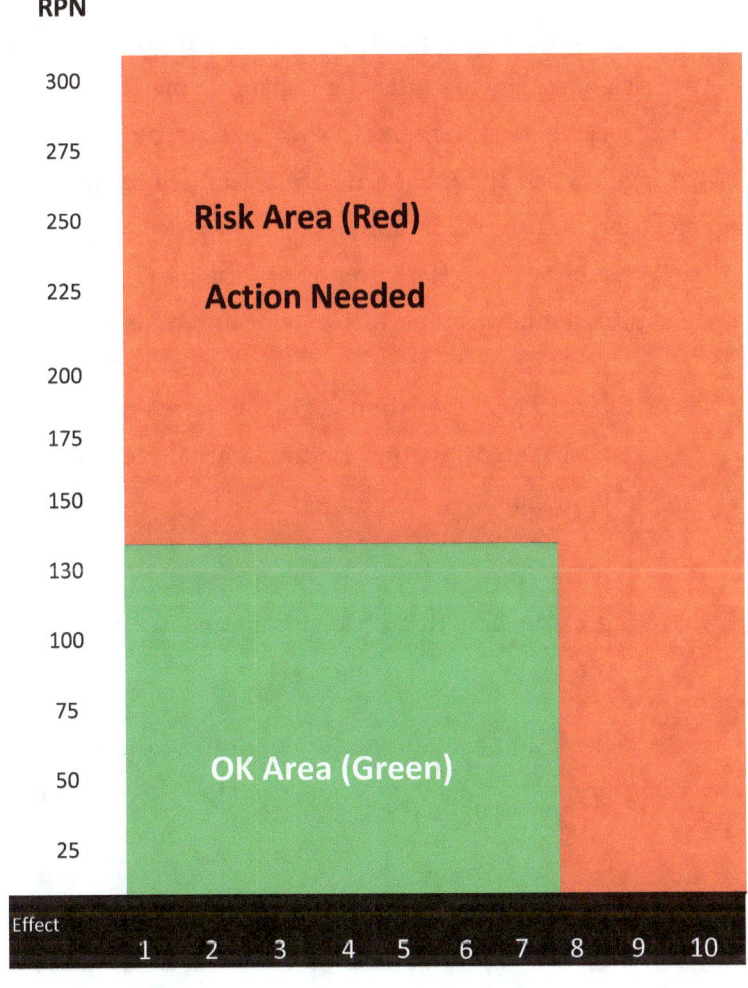

5.9 Rating RPN (second rating/option)

Once the measures have been identified in the first assessment, a second assessment will be carried out. which is an option and not a must. This means that we prepare the risk assessments after the registered measures such as IQ,OQ have been entered. Now let's think about what happens when the measures are actually implemented. In most cases, the risk is minimized, so the RPN is below the risk number we set. Here are the criteria for the second RPN (see p.61 template steps 12 to 16 for an option):

- If a RPN higher than 125 is achieved in the second assessment, further risk mitigation measures must be defined.

- If the impact number is equal to 8 and the RPN is greater than 101, an assessment of the risk must be made.

- If the impact number is equal to 9 and the RPN is greater than 76, an assessment of the risk must be made.

- If the impact number is equal to 10 and the RPN is greater than 51, an assessment of the risk must be made.

Table 5: Definition and evaluation of RPN **after** implementation of measures

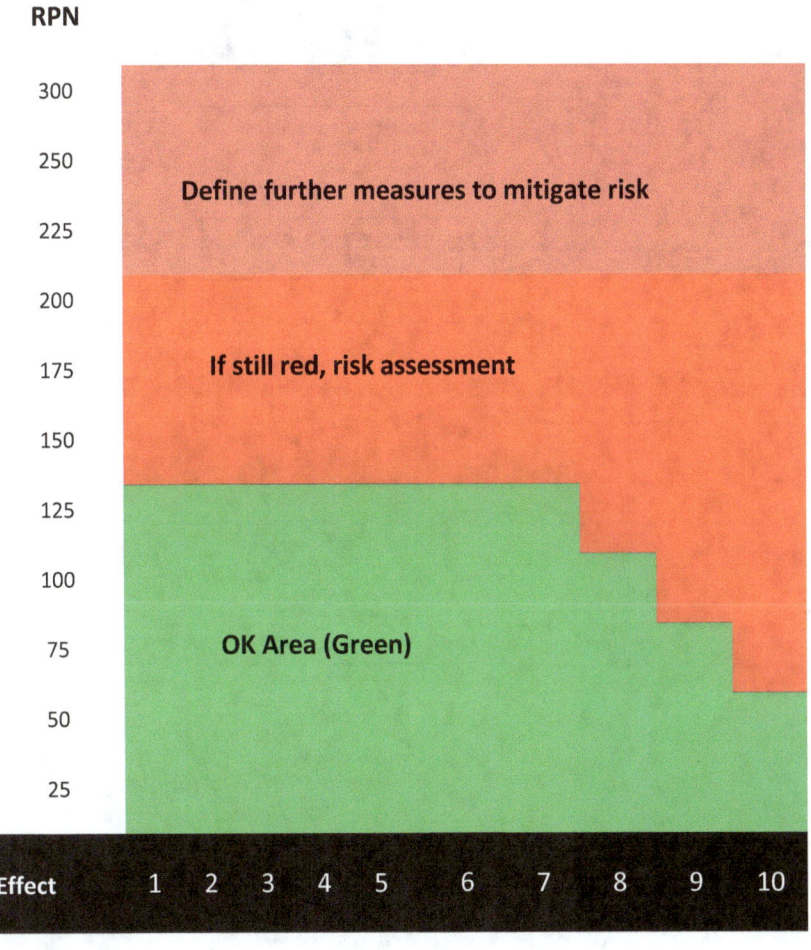

6. FMEA Process Flowchart

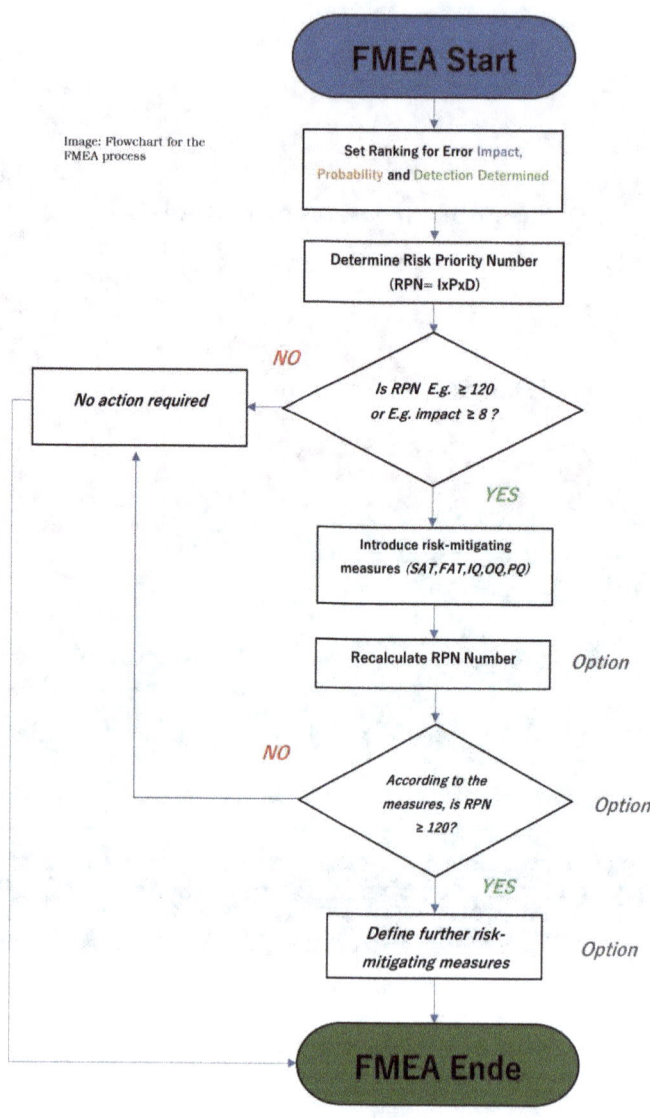

Image: Flowchart for the FMEA process

FMEA Start

Set Ranking for Error Impact, Probability **and** Detection Determined

Determine Risk Priority Number (RPN= IxPxD)

No action required

NO

Is RPN E.g. ≥ 120 or E.g. impact ≥ 8 ?

YES

Introduce risk-mitigating measures *(SAT,FAT,IQ,OQ,PQ)*

Recalculate RPN Number

Option

NO

According to the measures, is RPN ≥ 120?

Option

YES

Define further risk-mitigating measures

Option

FMEA Ende

42

7. FMEA Steps

1
- Describe possible relevant errors

2
- What can happen as a result of the error? Describe and enter the error effect number.

3
- Describe the reason for the error and enter the error probability number.

4
- How can the error be detected? Describe and enter the error detection number.

5
- Multiply the numbers from Impact & Probability & Detectability and enter them in the RPN column.

6
- w compare RPN figure with definition and evaluation table and determine a measure depending on the risk status.

option
- To reduce any risk, steps 2, 3, 4, 5 and 6 are repeated. (Definition and evaluation of the risk priority number after introduction of the measures)

8. FMEA Case Studies/Template

8.1 Project FMEA (Case Study No. 1)

Task: Project FMEA (for project implementation)

Project: Construction of a new production line for making ointment.

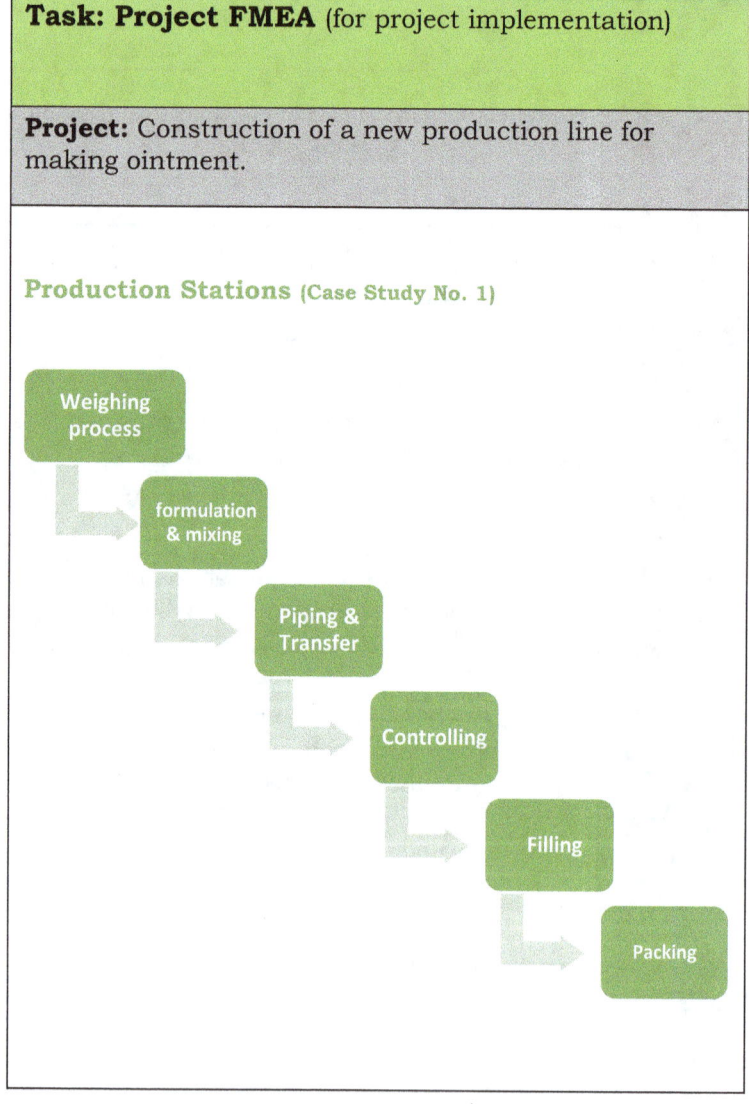

Production Stations (Case Study No. 1)

- Weighing process
- formulation & mixing
- Piping & Transfer
- Controlling
- Filling
- Packing

Case Study No. 1: Project Production Ointment / Production Stations

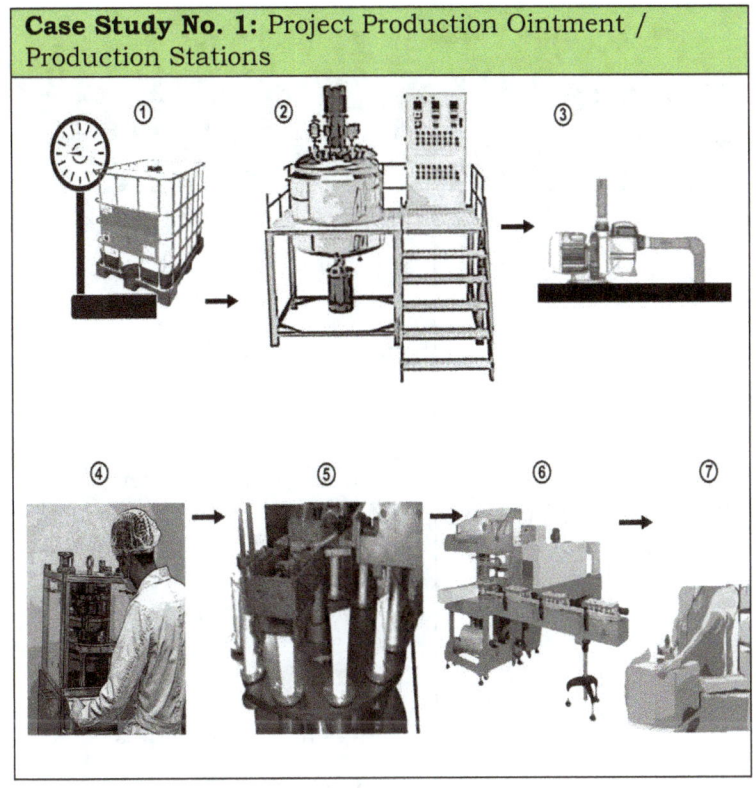

Task: Describe FMEA (Case Study No. 1)	
FMEA Steps (According to page 43/ Please pay attention to the color)	**As a possible answer for Production realization** (See Illustration No. 7)
FMEA Step❶ **Describe the possible project implementation errors:** See Illustration 10/Column 3	a-Delay in building conversion/dismantling b-Delay in acceptance by authorities c-Failure to meet delivery deadlines d-Incorrect deliveries e-Inconsistencies/malfunctions in other production lines during rebuild and so on..........
FMEA Step❷ **What can happen as a result of the errors?** See	a-Project costs can be increased b-Project realization in arrears/ endangered, ...

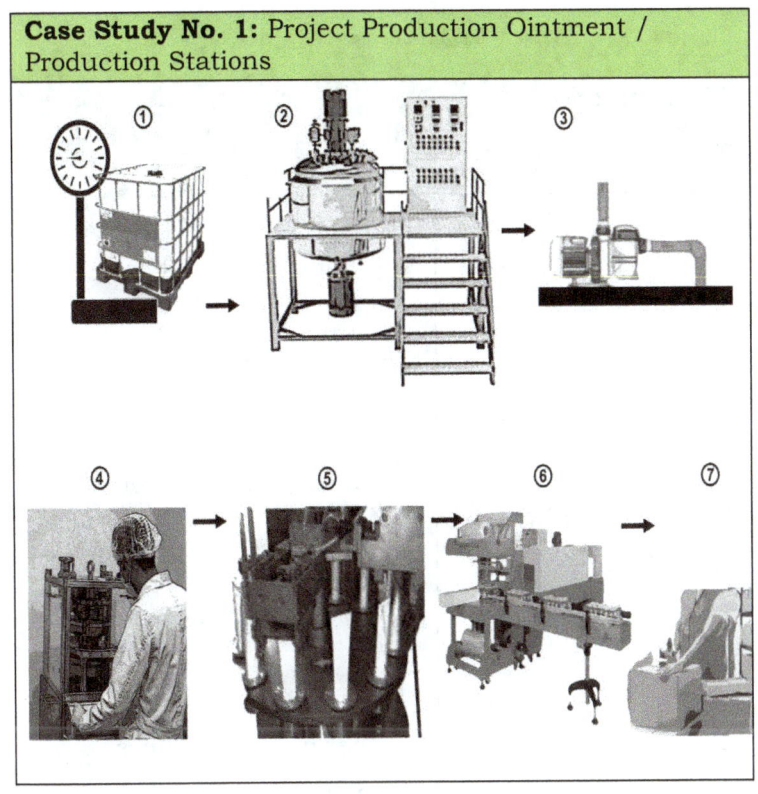

Task: Describe FMEA (Case Study No. 1)	
FMEA Steps (According to page 43/ Please pay attention to the color)	**As a possible answer for** **Production realization** (See Illustration No. 7)
FMEA Step❶ **Describe the possible** **project** **implementation** **errors:** See Illustration 10/Column 3	a-Delay in building conversion/dismantling b-Delay in acceptance by authorities c-Failure to meet delivery deadlines d-Incorrect deliveries e-Inconsistencies/malfunctions in other production lines during rebuild and so on..........
FMEA Step❷ **What can happen as** **a result of the** **errors?** See	a-Project costs can be increased b-Project realization in arrears/ endangered, ...

Illustration 10/Column 4+5	c-Project implementation in arrears/ endangered, ... d- Project implementation in arrears/ endangered, ... e- Total production stop and so on..........
FMEA Step❸ **Describe the potential cause of the error and enter the error probability number** See Illustration No. 10/Column 6+7	a-Internal approvals not yet completed / Budget not yet approved b-Necessary Documents not submitted/discrepancies c-Payments not yet made d-Supplier errors / Missing on-site inspections e- Lack of planning/lack of exchange of restructuring measures between departments and so on..........

FMEA Step❹	a- By supervisor/project manager
How can errors be detected? Describe and enter the error detection number. See Illustration 10/Columns 8+9	b- By supervisor/project manager
	c- By supervisor/project manager
	d- Through on-site inspections
	Project Manager/Coordinator
	and so on..........
FMEA Step❺	See Illustration 10/Column 10
Multiply numbers from Impact + Probability + Detectability and enter them in the RPN column.	

## FMEA Step ❻ **Now compare RPN number with definition and valuation table and define a measure depending on the risk level.**	See Illustration 10/Column 11
# Step Option: **To reduce any risk, steps 2, 3, 4, 5 and 6 are repeated. (Definition and evaluation of the risk priority number after the introduction of the measures)**	See Illustration No. 10/ Columns 12-16

Project FMEA

Ointment production project

Document No.: xxxx

Written by:

Role	Name	Title	Signature	Date
Author	Parviz Bayegi	QA-Engineer		

The author has created the document and confirms with its signature the substantive correctness

Reviewed and Approved by:

Roles	Name	Title	Signature	Date
Technical Reviewer	xxxxxxxxxx			
Process Owner	xxxxxxxxxx			
Technical Reviewer	xxxxxxxxxx			

The above-mentioned persons have checked this document and confirm with their signature the accuracy of the requirements

Document release by:

Role	Name	Title	Signature	Date
QA-Manager	Xxxx			

The QA Process Manager has reviewed the document, confirms the accuracy of the content with regard to quality compliance and regulatory requirements, and releases the document.

Illustration No. 8: Case study project FMEA (document name xx page 2 of x)

History of the document

Version / Datum	Reason for creation/modification
1.0 / Date	Re-creation as part of the project ....

Co-Applicable Documents

Dok.-Nr.	Title
XXXXXXXXXXXX	XXXXXXXXXXXXXX

51

TABLE OF CONTENTS

Explanations:

Point 1 Objective, subject matter and scope: all information about the project project and scope are explained here.

Point 2 General preliminary remarks: all FMEA preparations and assessment methods (see chapters 5 & 6 of the book) are shown here.

Point 3 Risk analysis: all areas are listed and processed in an Excel spreadsheet as shown in Illustration no.10.

Illustration No. 10 Case study project FMEA (document name xx/FMEA part)

Company Logo

Page x of z
Doc.-nr.: xxxx
Version: 1.0

FMEA for Project Implementation (Case Study)

Column No.	Function or requirement	Possible potential malfunction	Potential impact of the error	Impact (Ranking No.)	Possible Potential cause of the error	Probability (Ranking No.)	Possible detection of the error by	Detection (Ranking No.)	RPN	Recommended action	Neu Auswirkung	Neu Wahrscheinlichkeit	Neu Erkennung	Neu RPN	Neue Risiken identifiziert
1	Planning and preparation	E.g.: Delay in building conversion/ dismantling.	E.g.: Project implementation on in arrears/ endangered.	e.g.: 7	E.g.: Internal approvals not yet completed / Budget not yet approved	e.g.: 7	E.g.: By supervisor/ project manager	e.g.: 3	147	E.g.: weekly status reports/ creation of to-do lists	7	1	1	7	Unnecessary
2		Delay in acceptance by authorities :	Project implementation on in arrears/ endangered. :	7	E.g.: Necessary Documents not submitted/discrepancies	7	By supervisor/ project manager	3	147	E.g.: weekly status reports/appointment of a coordinator for authorities	Option	Option	Option	Option	Option
3		Failure to meet delivery deadlines :	Project implementation on in arrears/ endangered. :	7	E.g.: Payments not yet made	6	By supervisor/ project manager	5	210	Enter fixed delivery dates in the specifications/ord er/creation of FAT,SAT	Option	Option	Option	Option	Option
4		Incorrect deliveries	Project implementati on in arrears/ endangered.	7	E.g.: Supplier errors / Missing on-site inspections	6	Through on-site inspections	5	210	creation of FAT,SAT	Option	Option	Option	Option	Option
5		Inconsistencies/malfunctions in other production lines during rebuild	Total production stop	8	E.g.: Lack of planning/lack of exchange of restructuring measures between departments	6	Through on-site inspections	5	240	weekly status reports/appointme nt of a coordinator for restructuring measures between departments	Option	Option	Option	Option	Option
6		and so on.........	and so on.........		and so on.........		and so on.........			and so on.........	Option	Option	Option	Option	Option

53

Task: Design-FMEA

Project: Planning new piping for gases, sterile air pressure and steam.

Project/Structures

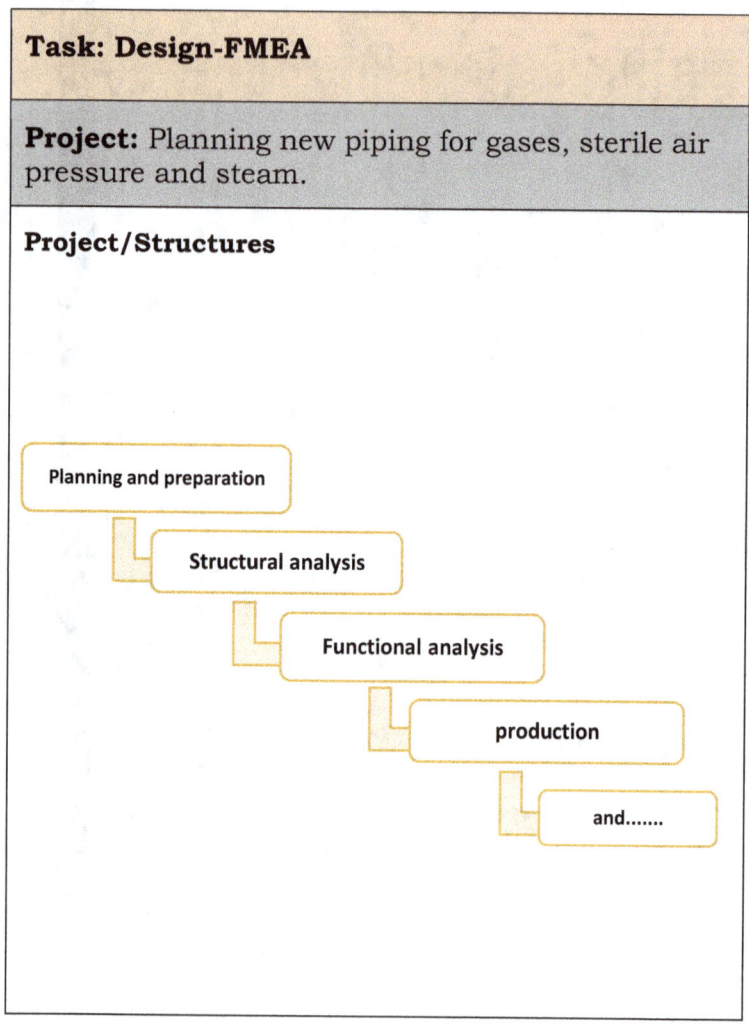

Company Logo	Page x of x
Design FMEA for the Project new Piping	Doc.-nr.: xxxx Version: 1.0

Design FMEA

Project new piping

Document No.: xxxx

Written by:

Role	Name	Title	Signature	Date
Author	Parviz Bayegi	QA-Engineer		
The author has created the document and confirms with its signature the substantive correctness				

Reviewed and Approved by:

Roles	Name	Title	Signature	Date
Technical Reviewer	xxxxxxxxxx			
Process Owner	xxxxxxxxxx			
Technical Reviewer	xxxxxxxxxx			
The above-mentioned persons have checked this document and confirm with their signature the accuracy of the requirements				

Document release by:

Role	Name	Title	Signature	Date
QA-Manager	Xxxx			
The QA Process Manager has reviewed the document, confirms the accuracy of the content with regard to quality compliance and regulatory requirements, and releases the document.				

Illustration No. 12 Case study Design-FMEA (document name xx/FMEA part)

1 Design-FMEA project for new lines

Column	1 Running No.	2 Function/ Requirement	3 Potential Error function	4 possible influence of the error	5 Impact (Ranking No.)	6 Potential Cause of the Error	7 Probability (Ranking No.)	8 Recognition	9 Recognition (Ranking No.)	10 RPN	11 Recommended action	12 New Impact	13 New Probability	14 New recognition	15 New RPN	16 New risks identified
	A	Planning and preparation	Unable to start scheduling	Project implementation in arrears/ endangered,...	e.g.:8	e.g.: Necessary Ifo. from the areas of manufacturing, quality, sales, service, marketing,	e.g.:6	By supervision / Project manager	e.g.:3	144	e.g.: Identify stakeholders, define project definition, create project charter; create work breakdown structure	8	2	1	16	Unnecessary
	B		Budget for the project not approved	Project realization in arrears/endan gered, further costs possible.	7	e.g.: Necessary documents not submitted/deviations present	6	By supervision / Project manager	3	126	e.g.: weekly status reports/appointment of a coordinator	Option	Option	Option	Option	Option
	C	Structural analysis	Integrity and security of planning not given	Project realization in arrears/endan gered, further costs possible.,...	8	e.g.: construction measures for the laying of pipelines have not been completed.	5	By supervision / Project manager	4	160	e.g.: create project charter, create work breakdown structure, weekly status reports,......	Option	Option	Option	Option	Option
	D	Functional analysis	Integrity at risk, quality checks not possible.	e.g.: Sampling of cables is not possible	8	e.g.: Plans are not prepared according to URS; review of plans was not possible	7	By supervision / Project Manager/ Acceptance	6	336	Have plans reviewed and approved	Option	Option	Option	Option	Option
	E	And more...														

56

8.3 Process-FMEA (Case Study No. 3)

Task: Process-FMEA

Project: Process validation production line for the production of ointments.

Process scope

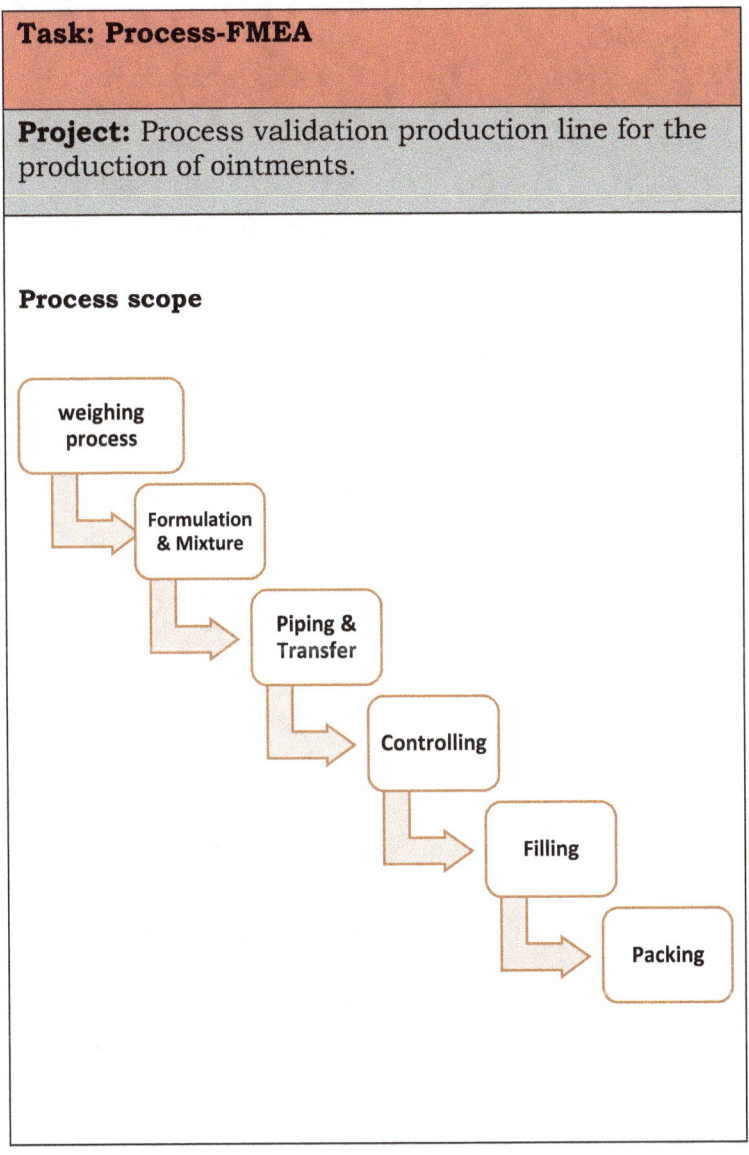

Case Study No. 3: Process-FMEA for the ointment production line (According to page 57)	
FMEA steps (According to page 43/ Please pay attention to the color)	**Possible answer for process**
FMEA Step❶ **Describe the possible errors during project implementation:** See Illustration No. 13/Column 3	A- e.g.: Quantities and weight deviations for raw materials For example: Containers are contaminated C- E.G.: Pipes are contaminated D- e.g.: Errors (wrong content, deviations) are not detected E-E.G.: Contamination during filling Q- E.G.: Wrong product or product with defect have been packaged

# FMEA Step❷ **What can happen as a result of the errors?** See Illustration 13/Columns 4+5	A- Formulation changes error, production stop B- Production stoppage/... C- Production stoppage/... D- Production stoppage/... E- Production stoppage/... F- Production stoppage/....
# FMEA Step❸ **Describe the potential cause of the error and enter the error probability number** See Illustration No. 13/Column 6+7	A- Uncalibrated balance, error in weighing protocol, B- Impure surface (of inner pipe) C- E.G.: due to dirt in the pipe D- e.g. control camera error, or control camera incorrectly positioned/installed

	E- e.g.: Hepa filter leaking
	F- Lack of control
## FMEA Step❹ **How can errors be detected? Describe and enter the error detection number.** See Illustration 13/Columns 8+9	A- By operators/QC staff B- By QA/QC staff C- By QA/QC staff D- By QA/QC staff E- By QA/QC staff F- By QA/QC staff
## FMEA Step❺ **Multiply numbers from Impact + Probability + Detectability and enter them in the RPN column.**	See Illustration 13/Column 10

8.3 Process-FMEA (Case Study No. 3)

Task: Process-FMEA

Project: Process validation production line for the production of ointments.

Process scope

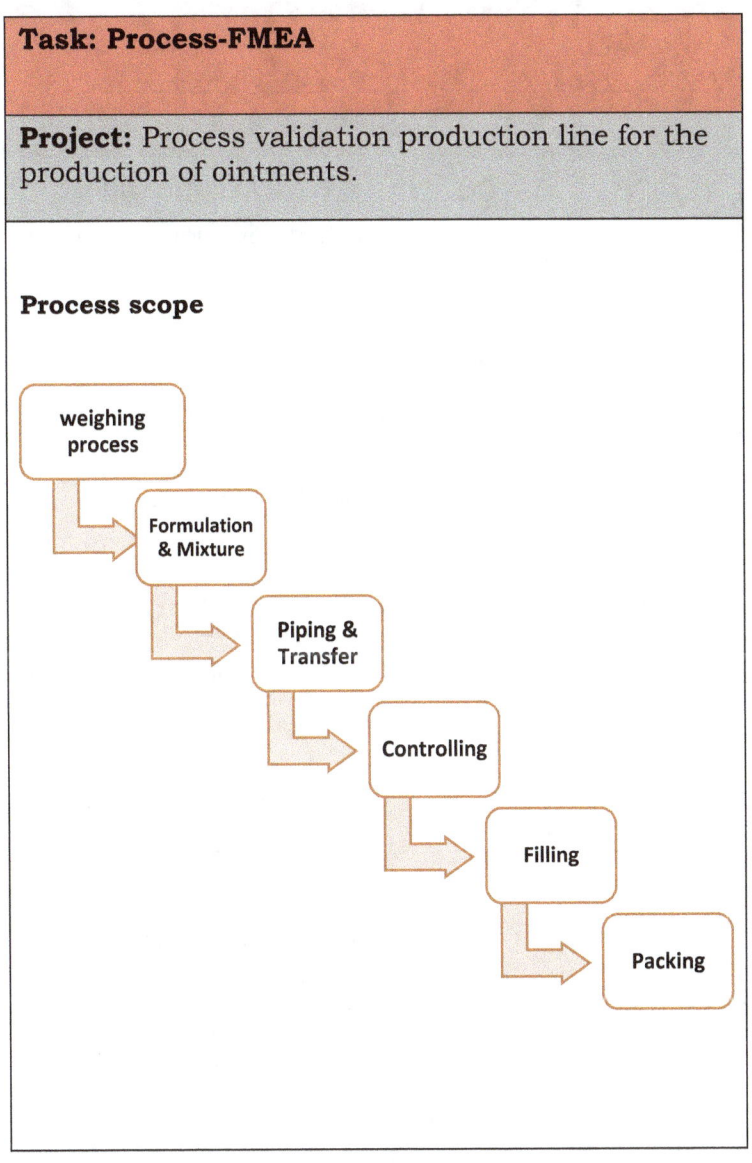

Case Study No. 3: Process-FMEA for the ointment production line (According to page 57)	
FMEA steps (According to page 43/ Please pay attention to the color)	**Possible answer for process**
FMEA Step❶ **Describe the possible errors during project implementation:** See Illustration No. 13/Column 3	A- e.g.: Quantities and weight deviations for raw materials For example: Containers are contaminated C- E.G.: Pipes are contaminated D- e.g.: Errors (wrong content, deviations) are not detected E-E.G.: Contamination during filling Q- E.G.: Wrong product or product with defect have been packaged

# FMEA Step ⑥ **Step Now compare RPN number with definition and valuation table and define a measure depending on the risk level.**	See Illustration 13/Column 11
# Step Option: To **reduce any risk, steps 2, 3, 4, 5 and 6 are repeated. (Definition and evaluation of the risk priority number after the introduction of the measures)**	See Illustration 13/See columns 12-16

Company Logo	Page x of x
Process FMEA	Doc.-nr.: xxxx Version: 1.0

Process FMEA for Project Ointment (Case Study)

Ointment production project

Document No.: xxxx

Written by:

Role	Name	Title	Signature	Date
Author	Parveez Baiegi	QA-Engineer		

The author has created the document and confirms with its signature the substantive correctness

Reviewed and Approved by:

Roles	Name	Title	Signature	Date
Technical Reviewer	xxxxxxxxxx			
Process Owner	xxxxxxxxxx			
Technical Reviewer	xxxxxxxxxx			

The above-mentioned persons have checked this document and confirm with their signature the accuracy of the requirements

Document release by:

Role	Name	Title	Signature	Date
QA-Manager	Xxxx			

The QA Process Manager has reviewed the document, confirms the accuracy of the content with regard to quality compliance and regulatory requirements, and releases the document.

Company Logo

Process FMEA case study

Col umn 1 Lfd. No.	2 Functi on or requir ement	3 Possible potential malfunction	4 Potential impact of the error	5 Impact (Ranking No.)	6 Possible Potential cause of the error	7 Probability (Ranking No.)	8 Possible detection of the error/by	9 Detection (Ranking No.)	10 RPN	11 Recommended action	12 New Impact	13 New Probability	14 New Detection	15 Or RPN	16 New risks / assess ed
A	Weighing process	E.g.: Quantities and weight deviations for raw materials	Formulatio n error, production stop	9	Scale not calibrated, error in weighing report,		By operators/Q C staff	7	315	Validated weighing process	9	3	1	27	Not necessary
B	Approach & Blend	E.g.: Containers are contaminated	Production stop/	9	Unclean surface	7	By QA/QC staff	7	441	Clean validation for batch technology and containers/SIP & CIP system validation	9	2	2	36	Not necessary
C	Piping & Transfer	E.g.: Pipes are contaminated	Production stop/	9	E.g.: due to dirt in the pipe	7	By QA/QC staff	6	378	Clean validation for the pipes/SIP & CIP system validation	9	2	1	18	Not necessary
D	Controlling	E.g.: Errors (wrong content, deviations) are not detected	Production stop/	9	E.g.: Camera error. Or camera incorrectly positioned/installe d	7	By QA/QC staff	6	378	Validate control system	9	2	1	18	Not necessary
E	Filling	E.g.: Contamination during filling	Production stop/	9	E.g.: Hepa filter leaking	6	By QA/QC staff	8	432	Validated monitoring for air flow/differentiatio n pressure/air particle measurement	9	1	1	9	Not necessary
F	Packing	E.g.: Wrong product or product with defect have been packaged	Production stop/	9	Lack of control	6	By QA/QC staff	7	378	Validated packaging process	9	1	1	9	Not necessary

Tabelle: Beispiel für ein FMEA Template

	1	2	3	4	5	6	7	8	9	10	11	12	13	14	15	16
Lfd. Nr.	Funktion/ Anforderung	Potentielle Fehl-funktion	Mögliche Einfluss des Fehlers	Auswirkung	Potentielle Ursache des Fehlers	Wahrscheinlichkeit	Erkennung	Erkennung	RPN (RPZ)	Empfohlene Maßnahme	Neu Auswirkung	Neu Wahrscheinlichkeit	Neu Erkennung	Neu RPZ (RPN)	Neue Risiken identifiziert	
Reinraum/ Wände																
1.1.	Wände/ Räume/ Boden	Raumpläne entsprechen nicht (installierten Räumen) as built	Projektstop/ Produktionsstop	8	Lieferantenfehler	6	Durch Projektleiter/ QA-Manager	5	240	IQ	8	2	3	48	Keine	
1.2.		Boden ist nicht leicht zu reinigen	Schmutz Ansammlungen/ aufwendige Reinigung notwendig	7	Lieferantenfehler	7	Projektleiter	4	196	∞	7	2	3	42	keine	
1.3.																

Erklärung zu den Spalten von FMEA Template

Spalt		Spalt		Spalt	
1	Laufende Nummer	7	Trage hier eine Zahl (1-10) aus der Bewertungsleitfaden für die Fehlerwarscheinlichkeit (S. 71)	15	Neue RPN wie Spalt 10 ermitteln
2	Anforderungen/Funktionen gemäß URS/Lastenheft	8	Sollte diese Fehler stattfinden, wie oder durch wer kann diese Fehler erkannt werden?	16	Ist eine neue Maßnahme nötig?
3	Der Wahrscheinliche Fehler bei dieser Anforderung/Funktion	9	Trage hier eine Zahl (1-10) aus der Bewertungsleitfaden für die Fehlererkennung (S. 72)		
4	Was passiert, wenn dieser Fehler vorkommt?	10	Durch Multiplikation von Auswirkungszahl x Wahrscheinlichkeitszahl x Erkennungszahl die RPN ermitteln		
5	Trage hier eine Zahl (1-10) aus dem Bewertungsleitfaden für die Fehlerauswirkung (S. 69) ein	11	RPZ Nummer mit dem Risikobereich aus der Tabelle (S. 77) vergleichen. Wenn RPZ eine Maßnahme zu der Minimierung von Risiko (GMP-Risiko) vorschreibt, dann diese hier eintragen	12,13,14	Angenommen, die Maßnahme (Nr. 11) zur Risikominimierung wurde durchgeführt. Wie würden Sie das Risiko nun bewerten? Um diesen Punkt neu zu bewerten, werden erneut in 12, 13 und 14 die Auswirkung, Wahrscheinlichkeit und Erkennung bewertet.
6	Was könnte die Ursache für den Fehler sein?				

Illustration No. 14: Case study process FMEA document/FMEA part

Process FMEA case study

Col umn	Lfd. No.	Function or requirement	Possible potential malfunction	Potential impact of the error	Impact (Ranking No.)	Possible Potential cause of the error	Probability (Ranking No.)	Possible detection of the error by	Detection (Ranking No.)	RPN	Recommended action	New Impact	New Probability	New Detection	Or gr.	New risk minimised
	2	3	4	5	6	7	8	9	10	11	12	13	14	15	16	
A	Weighing process	E.g.: Quantities and weight deviations for raw materials	Formulation error, production stop	9	Scale not calibrated, error in weighing report,	5	By operators/Q C staff	7	315	Validated weighing process	9	3	1	27	Not necessary
B	Approach & Blend	E.g.: Containers are contaminated	Production stop/	9	Unclean surface	7	By QA/QC staff	7	441	Clean validation for batch technology and containers/SIP & CIP system validation	9	?	2	36	Not necessary
C	Piping & Transfer	E.g.: Pipes are contaminated	Production stop/	9	E.g.: due to dirt in the pipe	7	By QA/QC staff	6	378	Clean validation for the pipes/SIP & CIP system validation	9	?	1	18	Not necessary
D	Controlling	E.g.: Errors (wrong content, deviations) are not detected	Production stop/	9	E.g.: Camera error. Or camera incorrectly positioned/installed	7	By QA/QC staff	6	378	Validate control system	9	2	1	18	Not necessary
E	Filling	E.g.: Contamination during filling	Production stop	9	E.g.: Hepa filter leaking	6	By QA/QC staff	8	432	Validated monitoring for air flow/differential pressure/air particle measurement	9	1	1	9	Not necessary
F	Packing	E.g.: Wrong product or product with defect have been packaged	Production stop/	9	Lack of control	6	By QA/QC staff	7	378	Validated packaging process	9	1	1	9	Not necessary

63

Illustration No. 15: FMEA table with explanations

Tabelle: Beispiel für ein FMEA Template

Lfd. Nr.	Funktion/ Anforderung	Potentielle Fehl-funktion	Mögliche Einfluss des Fehlers	Auswirkung	Potentielle Ursache des Fehlers	Wahrscheinlichkeit	Erkennung	Erkennung	RPN (RPZ)	Empfohlene Maßnahme	Neu Auswirkung	Neu Wahrscheinlichkeit	Neu Erkennung	Neu RPZ (RPN)	Neue Risiken identifiziert
1.1.	**Reinraum/ Wände**														
1.2	**Wände/ Räume/ Boden**	Raumpläne entsprichen nicht as built (installierten Räumen)	Projektstop/ Produktionsstop	8	Lieferantenfehler	6	Durch Projektleiter/ QA-Manager	5	240	IO	8	2	3	48	Keine
1.3		Boden ist nicht leicht zu reinigen	Schmutz Ansammlung/ aufwendige Reinigung notwendig	7	Lieferantenfehler	7	Projektleiter	4	196	OO	7	2	3	42	ke ne

Erklärung zu den Spalten von FMEA Template

Spalt		Spalt		Spalt	
1	Laufende Nummer	7	Trage hier eine Zahl (1-10) aus der Bewertungsleitfaden für die Fehlerwarscheinlichkeit (S. 71)	15	Neue RPN wie Spalt 10 ermitteln
2	Anforderungen/Funktionen gemäß URS/Lastenheft	8	Sollte diese Fehler stattfinden, wie oder durch wer kann diese Fehler erkannt werden?	16	Ist eine neue Maßnahme nötig?
3	Der Wahrscheinliche Fehler bei dieser Anforderung/Funktion	9	Trage hier eine Zahl (1-10) aus der Bewertungsleitfaden für die Fehlererkennung (S. 72)		
4	Was passiert, wenn dieser Fehler vorkommt?	10	Durch Multiplikation von Auswirkungazahl x Wahrscheinlichkeitszahl x Erkennungszahl die RPN ermitteln		
5	Trage hier eine Zahl (1-10) aus dem Bewertungsleitfaden für die Fehlerauswirkung (S. 69) ein	11	RPZ Nummer mit dem Risikobereich aus der Tabelle (S. 77) vergleichen. Wenn RPZ eine Maßnahme zu der Minimierung von Risiko (GMP-Risiko) vorschreibt, dann diese hier eintragen		
6	Was könnte die Ursache für den Fehler sein?	12,13,14	Angenommen, die Maßnahme (Nr. 11) zur Risikominimierung wurde durchgeführt. Wie würden Sie das Risiko nun bewerten? Um diesen Punkt neu zu bewerten, werden erneut in 12,13 und 14 die Auswirkung, Wahrscheinlichkeit und Erkennung bewertet.		

9. Glossar

DQ	Design Qualification
FAT	Factory Acceptance Test
FMEA	Failure Mode and Effect Analyse
GMP	Good Manufacturing Practice
IQ	Installation Qualification
OQ	Operation Qualification
PQ	Performance Qualification
RPN	Risk priority number
SAT	Site Acceptance Test
URS	User-Requirements-Specification

10. Quelle

GMP guidelines and associated appendices, especially Annex 15

ICH guideline Q9 on quality risk management EMA/CHMP/ICH

FDA guidelines and related appendices

GAMP (Good Automated Manufacturing Practice)

ISO 9001/ISO 14971/ISO13485-2016

Notiz:

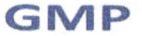 **GMP**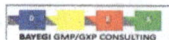

GMP -/FDA- Cleanroom planning & pharmaceutical engineering with practical case studies for

GMP

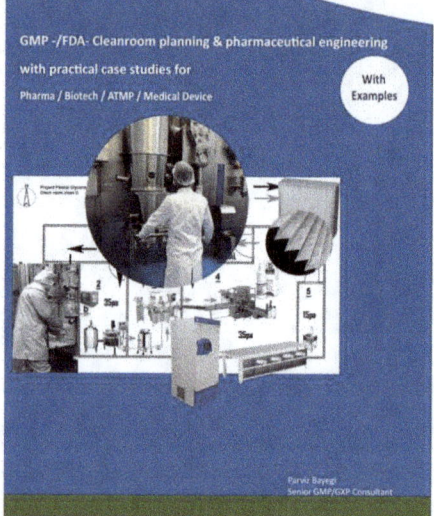

Topics in this book:

-Cleanroom standard/ ISO 14644

-Guidelines (GMP, FDA, PICs) for cleanroom production

-ISO/Standards for cleanroom construction

-GMP cleanroom construction and design

-Cleanroom construction/ components

-Ventilation technology in the cleanroom

-Cleanroom monitoring & measurements

-Materials & surfaces in the cleanroom

-Case study for the design of a GMP cleanroom

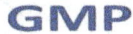 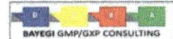 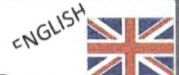

ENGLISH

GMP Compliance at Validation, Qualification & Docume
with practical case studies and templates for

Pharma / Biotech / ATMP / Medical Device   ISBN   978-1-4478-5510-1

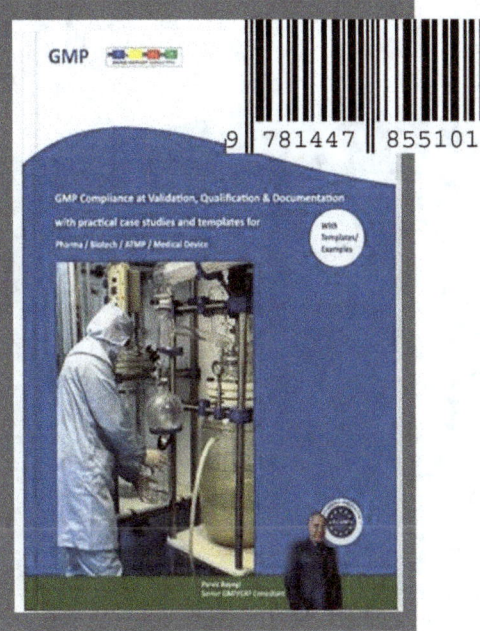

Topics in this book:

What is Qualification and what is Validation? Why do I qualify?

How do I get started with a GMP concept/project?

What are my GMP Qualification strategies?

How do I write a project risk analysis?

What is Change Control (CC) and do I need a Master or Sub CC?

How do I write a Validation Master Plan (VMP)?

What is a FMEA and why do I need a FMEA?

How do I write a FMEA? How do I write a Qualification plan (QP)?

What are FAT & SAT? And do I need these tests?

How do I create Qualification documents (DQ,IQ,OQ,PQ)?

Step by step to Validation and Qualification based on case studies

EU-GMP- Annex 1-2022
mit deutscher Übersetzung, Tipps und Hinweise

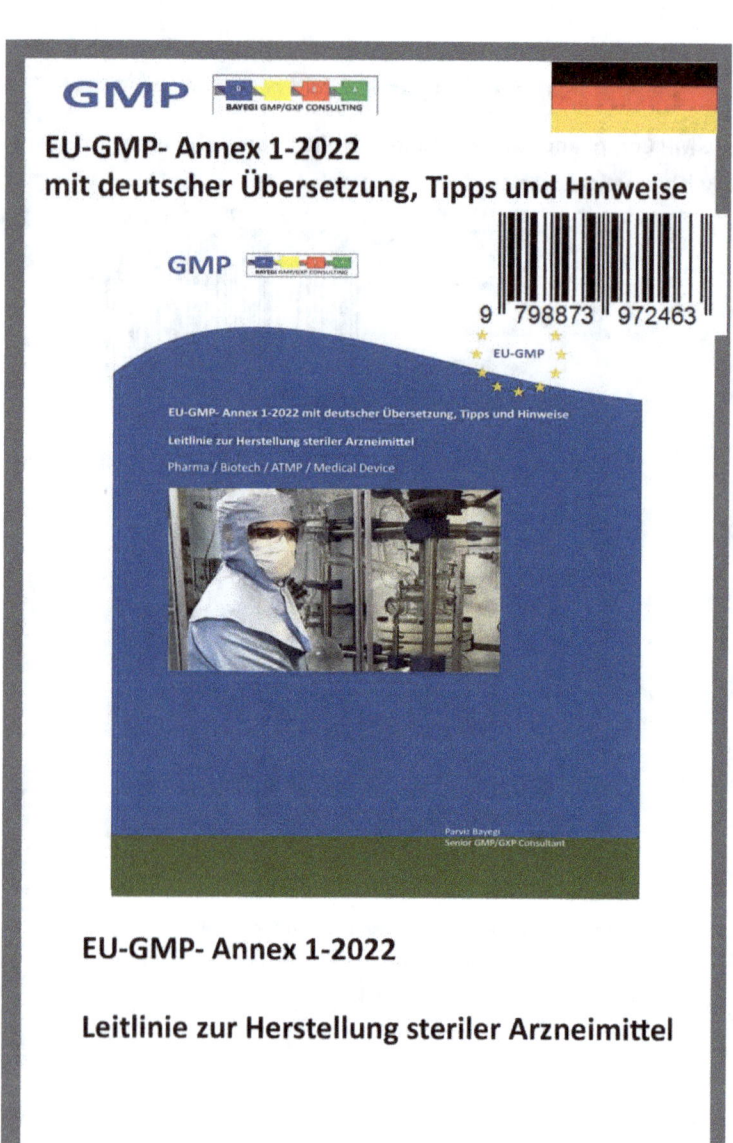

EU-GMP- Annex 1-2022

Leitlinie zur Herstellung steriler Arzneimittel

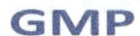 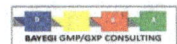

GMP- FAT & SAT Konzept und Durchführung

Mit praxisnahen Fallbeispielen und Template

für Pharma / Biotech / ATMP / Medical Device

 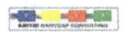

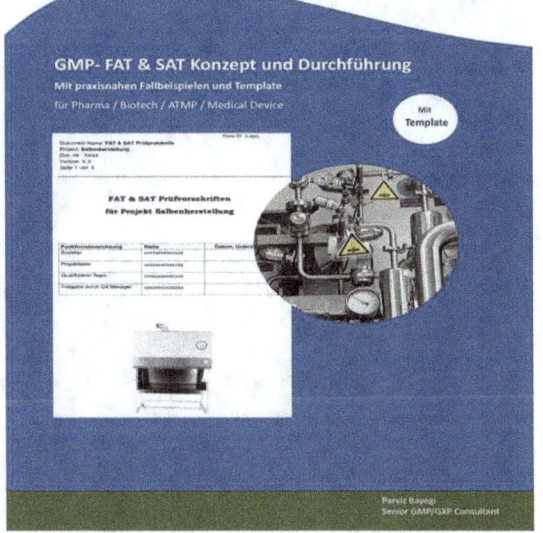

Themen in diesem Buch:

- Warum brauchen wir GMP-FAT/SAT?

- Besonderheiten von FAT & SAT bei GMP-Qualifizierung

- Wichtige FAT/SAT-Tests

- Implementierung in IQ & OQ

- FAT & SAT Konzept erstellen und schreiben

- Aufbau des Dokuments Prüfungsvorschriften

- Fallbeispiel für FAT/SAT-Dokumente

- Fallstudie FAT/SAT Prüfungen und Testprotokolle

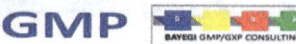

GMP- Lastenheft & Pflichtenheft für die Bestellprozesse

von Geräten & Anlagen innerhalb Reinräume und GMP-Projekten

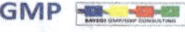

9 783347 902824

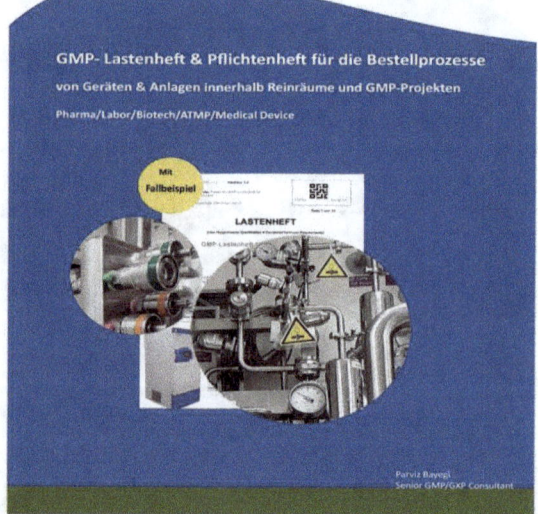

Themen in diesem Buch:

- Bestellprozesse & Dokumentierung bei GMP-Reinraumprojekten

- Allgemeine Anforderungen für GDP- & GMP-Dokumente

- GMP-Lastenheft und Qualifizierung

- Vorbereitung für GMP-Lastenheft

- URS

- Bestandteile eines GMP-Lastenheft & Pflichtenheft

- Schreiben eines GMP-Lasterhafts anhand eines Fallbeispiels

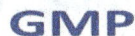 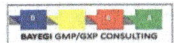

GMP- Kalibrierungen & SOP-Kalibrierungsdokumente

für Pharma / Biotech / ATMP / Medical Device

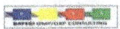

9 783347 898776

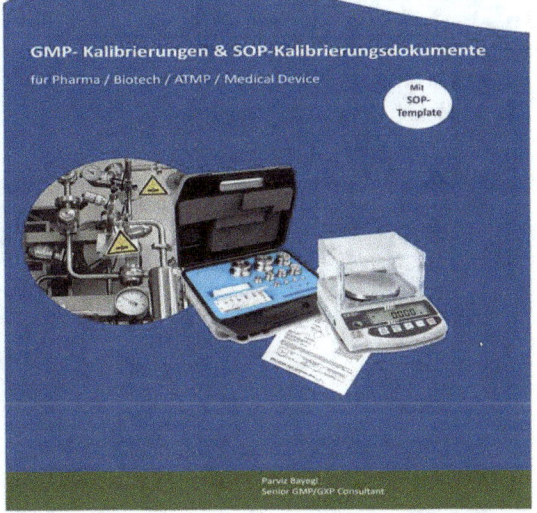

Themen in diesem Buch:

-Kalibrierung in Pharma/Labor

-Welche Normen gibt es für die Kalibrierung?

-Was bedeutet Kalibrierung, Justierung und Eichung

-Kalibrierungsarten

-Kalibrierungsintervall in GMP-Umgebung

-Wie wichtig ist eine Akkreditierung für ein Kalibrierungservice-Unternehmen?

-Welche Inhalte sollte ein Kalibrierschein in GMP-Umgebung haben?

-Wie wichtig ist die Rückverfolgbarkeit von Kalibrierungsnachweisen?

-Kalibrierungen Inhaus oder Extern?

-Aufbau einer SOP für Kalibrierungen

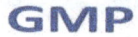 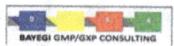 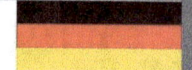

GMP-/FDA- Reinraumplanung & Pharma-Engineering

für Pharma / Biotech / ATMP / Medical Device

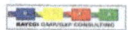

9 783347 883086

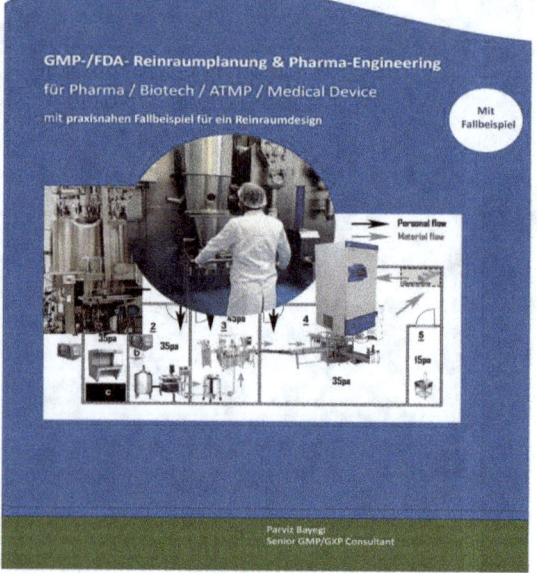

Themen in diesem Buch:

- Reinraum-Standardisierungen
- Richtlinien (GMP, FDA, PICs) für die Produktion im Reinraum
- ISO/Normen für den Reinraumbau
- GMP-Reinraumbau und Design
- Reinraum- Gebäudebestandteile
- Lüftungstechnik im Reinraum
- Reinraum-Monitoring & Messungen
- Werkstoffe & Oberflächen im Reinraum
- Fallstudie für die Planung eines GMP-Reinraums

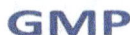 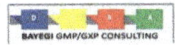 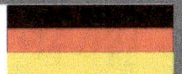

GMP- gerechte Validierung/Qualifizierung & Dokumentation
Mit praxisnahen Fallbeispielen und Templates für

Pharma / Biotech / ATMP / Medical Device

 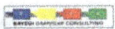 

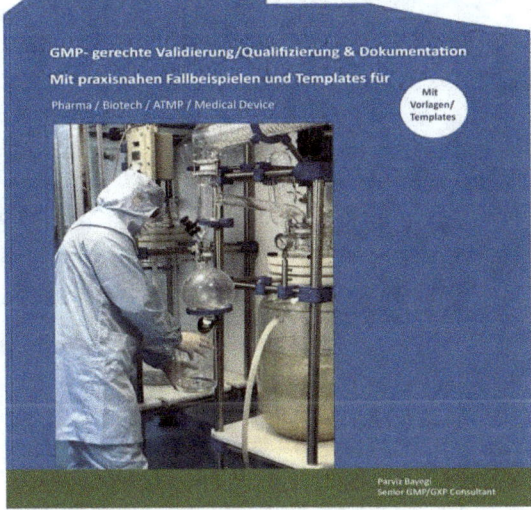

Themen in diesem Buch:

Was ist Qualifizierung und was ist Validierung?

Warum qualifiziere ich?

Wie beginne ich mit einem GMP-Konzept/Projekt?

Wie lauten meine GMP-Qualifizierungsstrategien?

Wie schreibe ich eine Projektrisikoanalyse?

Was ist Change control (CC) und brauche ich ein Master oder Sub CC?

Wie schreibe ich einen Validierungsmasterplan (VMP)?

Was ist ein FMEA und wozu brauche ich ein FMEA?

Wie schreibe ich ein FMEA?

Wie schreibe ich einen Qualifizierungsplan (QP)?

Was sind FAT & SAT? Und brauche ich diese Tests?

Wie erstelle ich Qualifizierungsdokumente (DQ,IQ,OQ,PQ)?

Schritt für Schritt zur Validierung und Qualifizierung anhand von Fallbeispielen

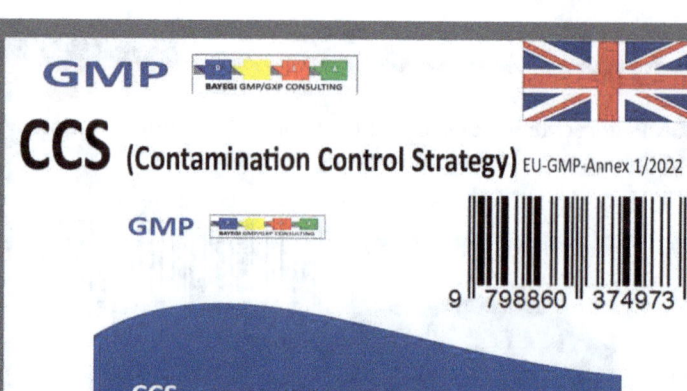

CCS (Contamination Control Strategy) EU-GMP-Annex 1/2022

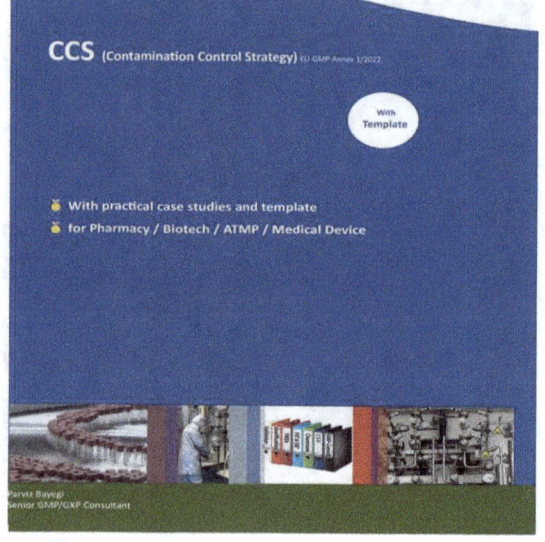

Topics in this book:

-QRM & CCS

-The Contamination Control Strategy (CCS) - What is it?

-How should a CCS umbrella document look like?

-What elements/areas does CCS contain?

-Example/template for CCS-Umbrella-Document

-Example/template for CCS excel list

-Internet Link for Template download

www.ingramcontent.com/pod-product-compliance
Lightning Source LLC
Chambersburg PA
CBHW071103290526

45795CB00004B/1632